# Welcome!

Are you excited to dive into some bodacious body love?

# Introduction

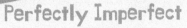

## Perfectly Imperfect

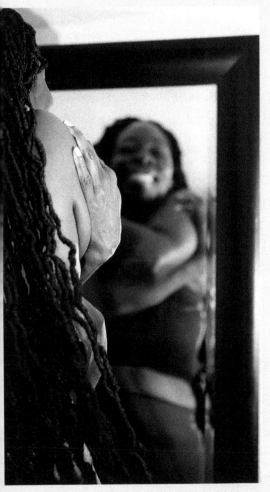

My fitness journey has been just that...perfectly imperfect.

I have tried it all to have the perfect body only to come to the realization that perfection is not what I initially thought it was. It is not the images I see on social media, the ones in my peer group, the one I imagine my favorite guy goes goo-goo ga ga over or even the image I close my eyes and wish to possess.

Instead, perfection, for me, is honoring what I see in the mirror because it is mine...intentionally selected by God for me! Perfection is being aware of how truly good my body has been to me. It is looking into the mirror and sometimes totally disliking what I see YET celebrating my perfectly imperfect body for what it is.. Yes, I'm talking about embracing my cellulite and loose skin because it's mine TOO!!!

My hope for you is that you too will come to learn, embrace and celebrate your body in all of its awesomeness.
My hope is you will learn to speak kind words to your body because it truly does hear you.

With bodacious body love,

Tysha

# How to use this journal

## 1

You're never alone! Meet your journal guide, Ty. IT is best to approach the journal in sequential order as each day builds on the previous day. At the start of each day she will provide you with prompts to get you started toward bodacious body love. Take your time, be open and journal freely for the best experience.

## 2

Truth makes us free but it can also upset us at first. At the end of each day you will have an opportunity to check in with yourself to bring awareness to your response to the day's entry. There will be space to note what led to your reaction and to brainstorm ways to move past it. if you choose.

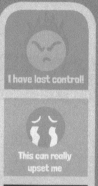

I have lost control!

This can really upset me

This can make me nervous

This bugs me

This never bothers me

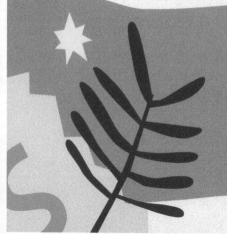

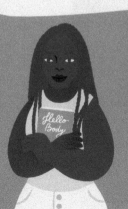

# Day One

Consider if you will your top three reasons for purchasing this journal. Have it in mind? THAT is your intention(s). It is your focused hope or goal. Once we identify an intention for ourselves it becomes pretty darn hard for anything to throw us off that focus. As you navigate through the next 21 days keep your intention(s) in mind. It is your intention(s) that open up the realm of possibilities inherent in this present experience. Today, spend time identifying and writing down your intention(s) for the experience.

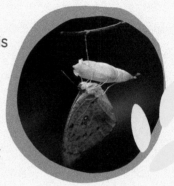

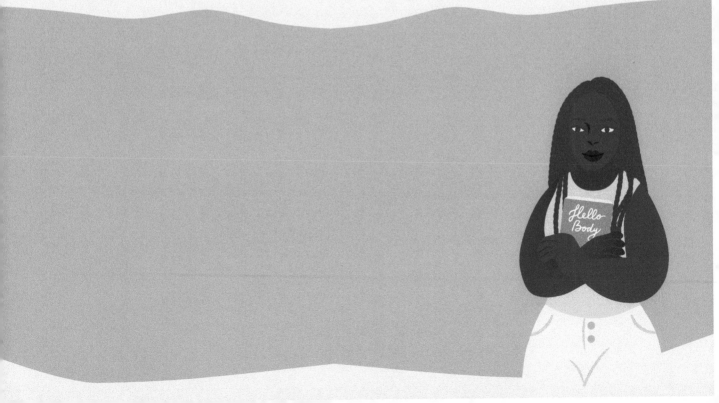

# Temperature Check

Rate how today's activity affected your mood.

If you are not where you'd like to be today, are there activities you may be able to engage in to assist you with improving your mood?

**HINT**:
Now would be a great time to add to your brag list.

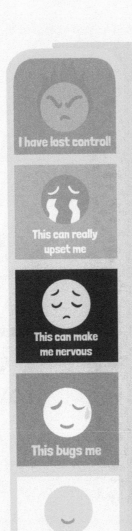

I have lost control!

This can really upset me

This can make me nervous

This bugs me

This never bothers me

# Day Two

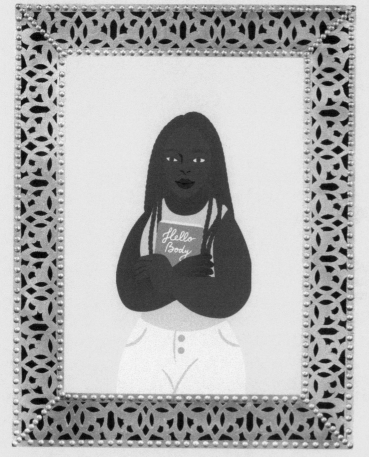

## Be Your Own Kind of Beautiful!

### Glue or tape a favorite picture of yourself here.

Today, describe what you like about your body on the following page. It's okay if you can not think of many, you can always come back to it.

# You can't help it that you're fabulous...

Don't be shy...develop a running list of all the fabulous things you love about your body. Add to your list daily. Commence to bragging NOW!!!

_____
_____
_____
_____
_____
_____
_____
_____
_____
_____
_____
_____
_____
_____
_____
_____
_____
_____
_____
_____
_____
_____
_____
_____

# Yup, I know you're fabulous... brag on :)

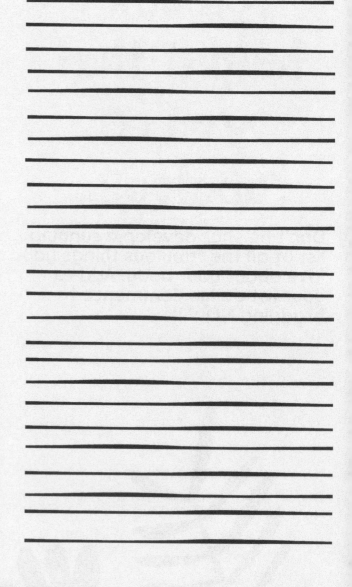

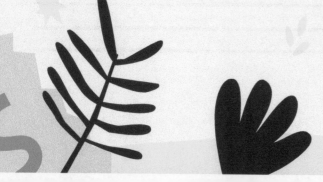

Notice your experience with today's activity.

Describe what went well and/or was challenging.

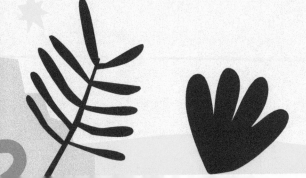

# Temperature Check

Rate how today's activity affected your mood.

If you are not where you'd like to be today, are there activities you may be able to engage in to assist you with improving your mood?

**HINT**:
Now would be a great time to add to your brag list.

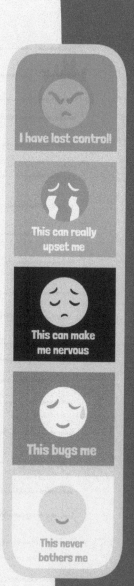

I have lost control!

This can really upset me

This can make me nervous

This bugs me

This never bothers me

# Day Three

Although our body is simply a mechanism or instrument that helps us interact with the world around us; the way we see, feel and relate to our body is what defines our body image.

Let's face it, every day is not the same. There are some days you may not be feeling your body as much as other days. A great thing to remember is it's just a day. You won't always feel this way and your body is not a determination of your value.

AND ALL OF THIS IS COMPLETELY NORMAL!!

Take some time today to just vent. What are the things you're just not feeling about your body TODAY!

Vent them below....noone is going to read this...allow yourself to be honest with yourself.

Do you notice any trends in your life? Are there thoughts about your body that come up more often? Are there moments you find more difficult to love your body? Describe them below.

# Temperature Check

Rate how today's activity affected your mood.

If you are not where you'd like to be today, are there activities you may be able to engage in to assist you with improving your mood?

**HINT**:
Now would be a great time to add to your brag list.

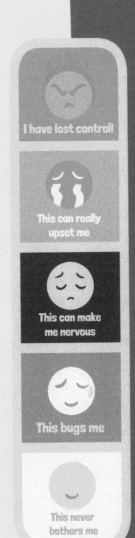

I have lost control!

This can really upset me

This can make me nervous

This bugs me

This never bothers me

# Day Four

Our brain is a beautiful thing!  It helps us navigate through life safely by creating internal messages (or thoughts) about our experiences.  Experiences can be direct or indirect, subtle or screaming loud!  An experience could be as simple as the look on someone's face when they glance at you or as big as the words or things a person says/does towards you.

Generally, if the experience was safe, our brain creates positive thoughts.  If the experience was threatening, our brain creates negative thoughts.

Whether safe or threatening those messages become cemented into our unconscious by becoming a part of our internal GPS navigation system.  Have you ever tried to drive to a destination with the wrong directions in your navigation system?  Challenging right?

In the same way, if you are attempting to move forward to bodacious body love with faulty navigation system directions you are going to get nowhere fast!!

Today, take a look at the messages you've received and how these messages help or hinder your movement towards body love.

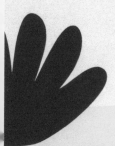

**What messages have I recieved from my family?**

_____
_____
_____
_____
_____
_____
_____
_____
_____
_____
_____
_____
_____
_____
_____
_____
_____

**What messages have I recieved from my friends?**

_____
_____
_____
_____
_____
_____
_____
_____
_____
_____
_____
_____
_____
_____
_____
_____
_____

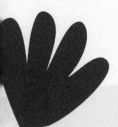

**What messages have I received from society?**

_____
_____
_____
_____
_____
_____
_____
_____
_____
_____
_____
_____
_____
_____
_____
_____
_____

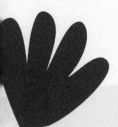
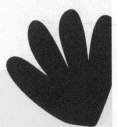

BE MORE SPECIFIC.
WHAT ARE THE MOST MEANINGFUL MESSAGES YOU'VE RECEIVED?

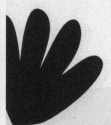

# Temperature Check

Rate how today's activity affected your mood.

If you are not where you'd like to be today, are there activities you may be able to engage in to assist you with improving your mood?

**\*\*HINT\*\*:**
Now would be a great time to add to your brag list.

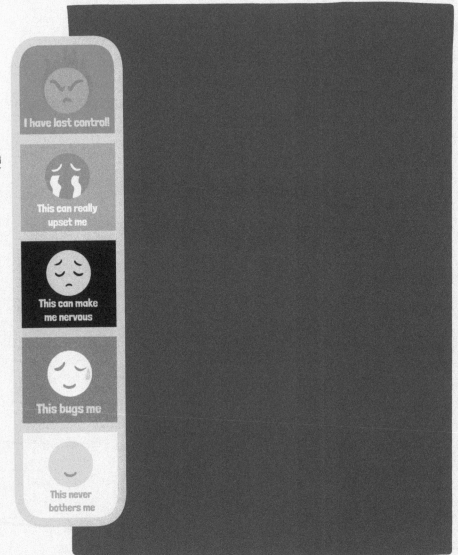

I have lost control!

This can really upset me

This can make me nervous

This bugs me

This never bothers me

# Day Five

Now that you have identified the various messages you have recieved,
consider how these messages shaped your beliefs, values and
expectaions about your body and self. How do they shape your what
you say to yourself about yourself?  Describe below.

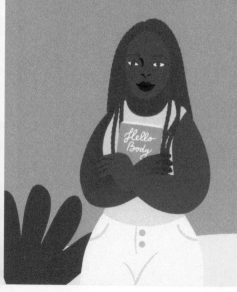

# Temperature Check

Rate how today's activity affected your mood.

If you are not where you'd like to be today, are there activities you may be able to engage in to assist you with improving your mood?

**HINT**:
Now would be a great time to add to your brag list.

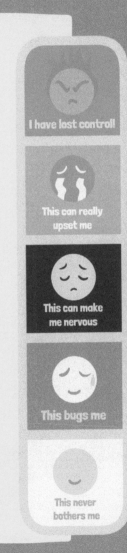

# Day Six

Say this with me: I am human, therefore I feel.
Okay, one more time for the people in the cheap seats!!

Feelings are a normal part of the human experience. They work alongside our thoughts as a part of our internal navigation system. Remember that childhood song: "first comes love, then comes marriage..."

Our feelings are responses to the internal messages (or thoughts) we hold. First comes thoughts, then comes feeling...

It's a chain reaction!

**A feeling is just a feeling!!**

Feelings can present themselves in varying intensities, as you likely noticed during your daily temperature check. Feelings can also be multi-faceted and complex. Some also describe their feelings as conflicting. Uncomfortable feelings can produce stress within our brain. As a result we may find ourselves in a natural stress response by fighting-running-or freezing. This would be why it feels so yucky to hold on to negative self talk.

Consider how much more helpful it would be to allow all of your feelings...the comfortable AND uncomfortable ones so you may become aware of what they are directing you to---your deeper needs. When we address our deeper needs we are able to release what no longer moves us forward.

Today, sort through your feelings. I've included a feelings cheat sheet if you need a reference. Which emotions do you experience most about your body? Where and how in your body do you experience these feelings?

Did you know: Science shows the lifetime of a feeling- from the initial psychiolological signs in the body to the time it resolves is 90 seconds. Hear that, NINETY seconds. What expands the life cycle of a feeling is our need to control the experience.

| | | | | | |
|---|---|---|---|---|---|
| Sure | Depressed | Uncertain | Amused | Annoyed | Determined |
| Certain | Desperate | Upset | Delighted | Agitated | Inspired |
| Unique | Dejected | Doubtful | Glad | Fed up | Creative |
| Dynamic | Heavy | Uncertain | Pleased | Irritated | Healthy |
| Tenacious | Crushed | Indecisive | Charmed | Mad | Renewed |
| Hardy | Disgusted | Perplexed | Grateful | Critical | Vibrant |
| Secure | Upset | Embarrassed | Optimistic | Resentful | Strengthened |
| Empowered | Hateful | Hesitant | Content | Disgusted | Motivated |
| Ambitious | Sorrowful | Shy | Joyful | Outraged | Focused |
| Powerful | Mournful | Lost | Enthusiastic | Raging | Invigorated |
| Confident | Weepy | Unsure | Loving | Furious | Refreshed |
| Bold | Frustrated | Pessimistic | Marvelous | Livid | |
| Determined | | Tense | | Bitter | |

# Temperature Check

Rate how today's activity affected your mood.

If you are not where you'd like to be today, are there activities you may be able to engage in to assist you with improving your mood?

**HINT**:
Now would be a great time to add to your brag list.

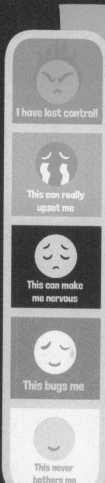

I have lost control!

This can really upset me

This can make me nervous

This bugs me

This never bothers me

# Day Seven

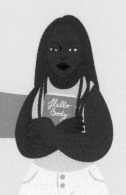

**fear** /ˈfir/ — Noun: an unpleasant, often strong emotion caused by anticipation or awareness of danger

## My deepest body fears are...

**FEAR 1**

**FEAR 2**

**FEAR 3**

Let's play your fears out.  If your deepest body fear
actually came true what would happen next?
What need is your fear directing you to?

What would having these things happen in your life mean for you? How realistic is this fear? Can you think of ways you would still be okay if your deepest body fear actually happended?  Describe below.

# Temperature Check

Rate how today's activity affected your mood.

If you are not where you'd like to be today, are there activities you may be able to engage in to assist you with improving your mood?

**\*\*HINT\*\*:**
Now would be a great time to add to your brag list.

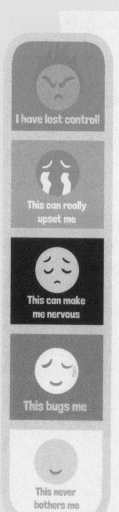

I have lost control!

This can really upset me

This can make me nervous

This bugs me

This never bothers me

# Day Eight

**Many times when we feel uncomfortable feelings about a thing we try unhelpful (or helpful) strategies to control our experience.**

- What has your feelings towards your body led you to do over the years?
- What impact has these actions had on your life?
- Are you happy with this impact?
- What would need to change to increase your happiness?
- What stops you from making these changes?
- What could you differently today?

*Thoughts are inevitable, behaviors are optional so choose wisely!*

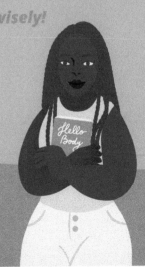

# Temperature Check

Rate how today's activity affected your mood.

If you are not where you'd like to be today, are there activities you may be able to engage in to assist you with improving your mood?

**HINT**:
Now would be a great time to add to your brag list.

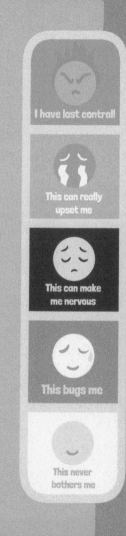

# Day Nine

Mindfulness is the intentional practice of becoming more aware of your present experience. It simply is keeping up with what is happening here and now.
Learning to be more mindful about your internal world is paramount to creating the experiences you desire.

Today, carve out 20 minutes to practice the following mindfulness activity. When complete, describe your experience. The more you practice mindfulness the better equipped you become at picking up on shifts in your mood created by inevitable thoughts.

Pick 3 songs from different genres and of varying tempos. Listen to each song paying attention to what you hear (the words, rhythm, tempo, etc). As you are listening also attend to how your body responds. Does your breath become shallow, more labored, do your palms become sweaty, do your muscles tighten, etc? Your body will clue you into which feelings you are experiencing.
What thoughts are connected to the feelings your body experienced?

Describe your experience.

Does your imagination wonder, it's okay to write down your thoughts and start over as many times as you need.

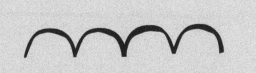

# Temperature Check

Rate how today's activity affected your mood.

If you are not where you'd like to be today, are there activities you may be able to engage in to assist you with improving your mood?

**\*\*HINT\*\*:**
Now would be a great time to add to your brag list.

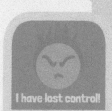

I have lost control!

This can really upset me

This can make me nervous

This bugs me

This never bothers me

# Day Ten

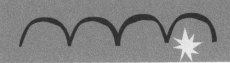

# Who's your judge?

A judgement is the decision we form based on data presented to us. This data could be our own or others. In both cases we get to choose whether we continue to own these judgements. Yes, you have the choice to reject even your own decisions by choosing differently at any time.

Using your mindfulness skills, think of a repetitive judgement(s) you hold about your body. Describe it in detail. How do these judgments make you feel? Do these judgements cause you to project your thoughts onto others? Do these judgements tempt you to predict the future? How so?
What's your go-to stress response when you feel judged by yourself?

The interesting thing is: it isn't necessarily the thought that causes us to experience big emotions, it is the judgements we hold about our experience that is most distressing to us.

# Temperature Check

Rate how today's activity affected your mood.

If you are not where you'd like to be today, are there activities you may be able to engage in to assist you with improving your mood?

**HINT**:
Now would be a great time to add to your brag list.

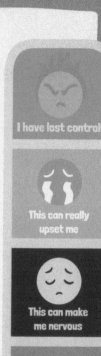

# Day Eleven

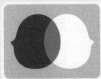

### BLACK AND WHITE THINKING
Believing that something or someone can be only good or bad, right or wrong, rather than anything in between or 'shades of grey'.

### CRITICAL SELF
Putting ourselves down, self-criticism, blaming ourselves for events or situation that are not (totally) our responsibility.

### EMOTIONAL REASONING
I feel bad so it must be bad! I feel anxious so I must be in danger.

### MENTAL FILTER
When we notice only what the filter allows or wants us to notices and we dismiss anything that doesn't 'fit'. Like looking through dark blinkers or 'gloomy specs', or only catching the negative stuff in our 'kitchen strainers' whilst anything more positive or realistic is dismissed.

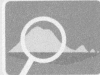

### MOUNTAINS AND MOLEHILLS
Exaggerating the risk of danger, or the negatives. Minimising the odds of how things are most likely to turn out, or minimising positives.

### SHOULDS AND MUSTS
Thinking or saying 'I should' (or shouldn't) and 'I must' puts pressure on ourselves, and sets up unrealistic expectations.

### MIND READING
Assuming we know what others are thinking (usually about us).

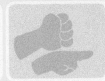

### JUDGEMENTS
Making evaluations or judgments about events, ourselves, others, or the world, rather than describing what we actually see and have evidence for.

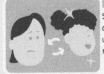

### COMPARE AND DESPAIR
Say only the good and positive aspects in others, and getting upset when comparing ourselves negatively against them.

### PREDICTION
Believing we know what's going to happen in future.

### MEMORIES
Current situations and events can trigger upsetting memories, leading us to believe that the danger is here and now, rather than in the past, causing us distress right now.

### CATASTROPHISING
Imagining and believing that the worst possible thing will happen.

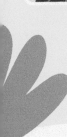

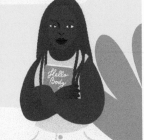

# Temperature Check

Rate how today's activity affected your mood.

If you are not where you'd like to be today, are there activities you may be able to engage in to assist you with improving your mood?

**HINT**:
Now would be a great time to add to your brag list.

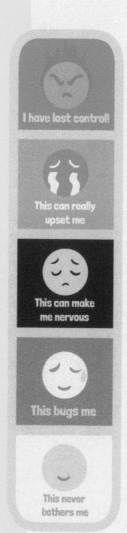

# Day Twelve

Further consider the judgements you discovered yesterday. What would life be like if you were less judgemental towards yourself? Learning to be less judgemental takes practice. It involves becoming aware of extreme ways of thinking that are not realistic. Today, let's look closer at your judgements. Are there extremes in your internal lanage. "right," "wrong," "fair," "unfair," "should," "shouldn't," "stupid," "lazy," "wonderful," "perfect," "bad," and "terrible."

Practice identifying your judgemental lanage.

**1**

When xyz happens...

I can not fit my cloting.

**2**

I tell myself...

I am fat and I will never have the perfect body.

**3**

My judgemental language is...

Never and Perfect because these are not realistic way of seeing myself.

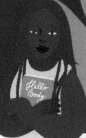

**1**

When xyz happens...

**2**

My judgemental lanagage is..

**3**

I can choose to tell myself...

# Now let's practice

**1**

When xyz happens...

**2**

My judgemental lanagage is..

**3**

I can choose to tell myself...

# Now let's practice

**1**

When xyz happens...

**2**

My judgemental lanagage is..

**3**

I can choose to tell myself...

# Temperature Check

Rate how today's activity affected your mood.

If you are not where you'd like to be today, are there activities you may be able to engage in to assist you with improving your mood?

**HINT**:
Now would be a great time to add to your brag list.

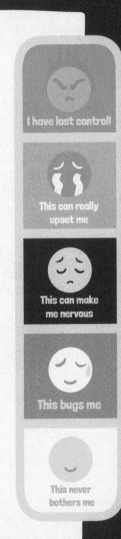

I have lost control!

This can really upset me

This can make me nervous

This bugs me

This never bothers me

# Day Thirteen

## Breathe 1... 2... 3...

Sometimes we can be overwhelmed in the moment which causes us to react out of our emotions rather than from a place of regulated, higher level thinking... where the good stuff is. To get to the good stuff, our brain has to calm all the way down. Breathing is THE answer!!! Breathing acts just like a fan to calm our brain down enough so that we are able to remain regulated and see things more clearly. Today, let's practice the skill of deep breathing. Take your time and practice 5-10 sets. Describe your experience when you are done.

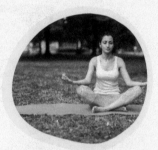

If deep breathing is new to you, find a space free from distractions. Position yourself comfortably.

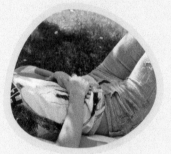

Put one hand on your belly just below your ribs and the other hand on your chest.

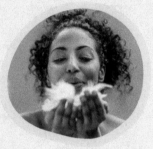

Take a deep breath in through your nose letting your belly rise an fall with your breath. Breathe out through your mouth.

# Temperature Check

Rate how today's activity affected your mood.

If you are not where you'd like to be today, are there activities you may be able to engage in to assist you with improving your mood?

**HINT**:
Now would be a great time to add to your brag list.

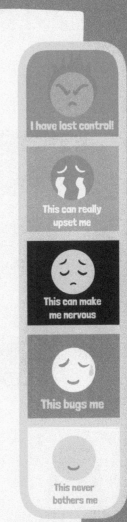

I have lost control!

This can really upset me

This can make me nervous

This bugs me

This never bothers me

# Day Fourteen

# You're coming out and letting go!

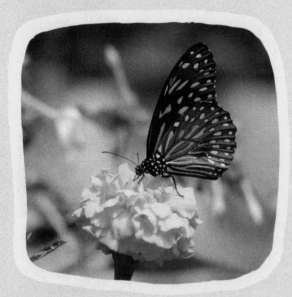

Sometimes, life has happened and we carry the weight of life on our body. The weight (overweight or underweight) is not simply a matter of pounds but of life experiences and how we've responded to those experiences.

Just like a butterfly trapped in its cocoon, when we hold on to an experience we also hold ourselves back from celebrating the true beauty and uniqueness of our real body. Let's flip that on its head today. Journal about what you're really holding on to and what would it mean to let that go.

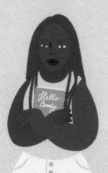

# Temperature Check

Rate how today's activity affected your mood.

If you are not where you'd like to be today, are there activities you may be able to engage in to assist you with improving your mood?

**HINT**:
Now would be a great time to add to your brag list.

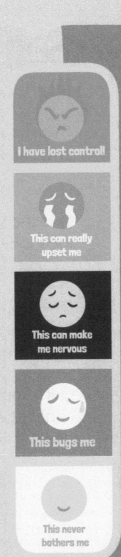

I have lost control!

This can really upset me

This can make me nervous

This bugs me

This never bothers me

# Day Fifteen

# My-Self-Love

Having "My-self-love" or self compassion is not about what others think or feel. It is about having an accurate understanding of yourself and then accepting yourself just as you are while you are on the way to where you want to be.

Even if someone is giving you their opinion of you it is there opinion born out of ther experiences, values and judgements. It does not have to be your own.

My-self-love involves silencing the voce of others-and sometimes your own inner critic- so that you see yourself with the eyes of grace and love. My-self-love means allowing your voice about you to be the loudest.

It could also mean setting boundaries around the things that create faulty standards for yourself- eliminating or reducing the amount of time spent engaging in those things.

My-self-love can also mean loving yourself enough to challenge yourself to grow and develop in a way greater than you currently are.

What I've come to realize is the more love I provided my body, the more my desire to care for it increased. Not with the intention to change it but with the intention to care and nourish it.

Question 1: How has your inner critic shown up in your life?

Question 2: What does My-self-love look like for you?

Question 2: How can you create boundaries in your life that promote My-self-love?

Question 2: How can you challenge yourself to grow in a greater way?

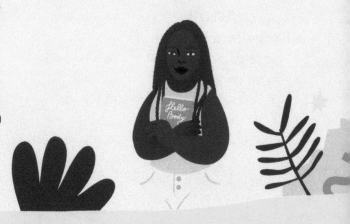

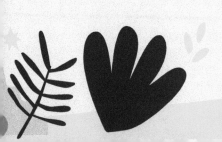

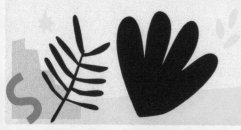

# Temperature Check

Rate how today's activity affected your mood.

If you are not where you'd like to be today, are there activities you may be able to engage in to assist you with improving your mood?

**HINT**:
Now would be a great time to add to your brag list.

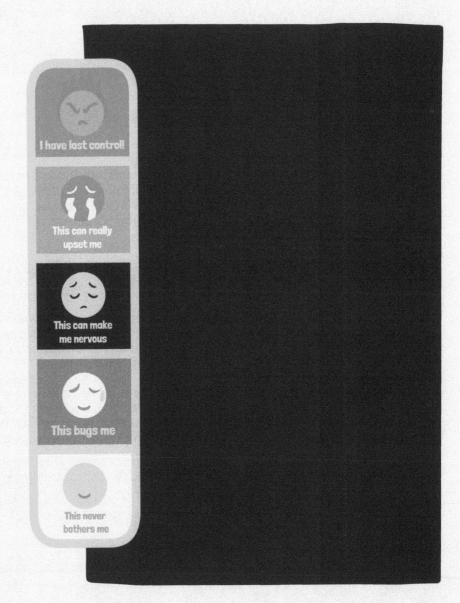

# Day Sixteen

## You are your own Standard!!

Standard: an idea or thing used as a measure, norm or model for evaluation purposes. When setting a standard one considers things such as our personal values , purpose and goals.  Your Creator gave you a purpose and intentionally crafted your body for the His intended purpose for you.  We are all unique in purpose then it would follow that we would be unique in our body's characteristics. To honor your uniqueness would be to honor your Creator.

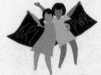

## A little sister to sister chat.

Listen, you do not have to always be happy about your body to accept and embrace it. Discontent is another very valid emotion.  All emotions are worth acknowledging. Positive body image isn't about perfection.  It is about having a true sense of self and your body.

What would it mean to you to accept there will be days where you are dissatisfied and it is completely normal.  You no longer have to struggle with that all or nothing thinking if you choose to practice not attempting to change or act on the things you are not able to change. It's okay to just let go of what you are not able to change.

Which of your personal values, purpose and goals have helped to create your body's standard? Do these values support positive body image? If not, how can you shift this for yourself, today?

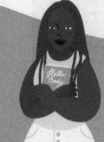

# Temperature Check

Rate how today's activity affected your mood.

If you are not where you'd like to be today, are there activities you may be able to engage in to assist you with improving your mood?

**HINT**:
Now would be a great time to add to your brag list.

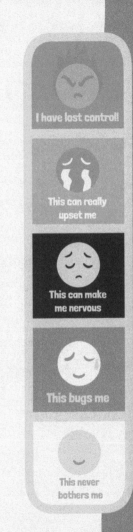

I have lost control!

This can really upset me

This can make me nervous

This bugs me

This never bothers me

# Day Seventeen
## It's a body-looza

Affirming your body does not have to be just about physical characteristics. It can be about what your body has allowed you to do, it's strength, power, poise, and endurance, for example.

Today, slow down and take time getting re-acquainted with your body. Below, describe characteristics of your body you may have never considered. If you need help, try this: write a body timeline of your body's life. You were born, which is a worthy body accomplishment in itself!! Did you also play sports, bare children, fight a medical issue, struggled with yo-yo dieting? Acknowledge your body's noted strengths and which challenges your body helped you overcome? This activity will move you forward on your journey.

# Temperature Check

Rate how today's activity affected your mood.

If you are not where you'd like to be today, are there activities you may be able to engage in to assist you with improving your mood?

**HINT**:
Now would be a great time to add to your brag list.

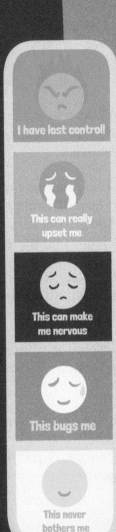

I have lost control!

This can really upset me

This can make me nervous

This bugs me

This never bothers me

# Day Eighteen
# YoUr WoRdS hAvE pOwEr!!

Have you ever realized your body is alive? As a living organism, your body has the ability to hear and respond. Your body has the capacity to grow, adapt and reproduce.

The world and everything in it listens and responds to the words we speak. I remember reading a study that spoke of how affirming words activate our brain's reward system. Essentially, the words we speak counters any stressful or threatening situation we are facing-including the negative thoughts we may think about our body.

As such, we were born with the creative capacity to shape our world. Imagine that!!! Change, body change, can begin by what I allow myself to speak.

We do not always responsibly use this super power we possess. More often, we spend our time speaking our worries and fears which is, perhaps, why we continue believing and experiencing what we speak.

Activate your superpower and watch how everything in your world shifts.

Today, practice using the power of your words to affirm the values and goals you have for your body.

**What you see...**

My body is ugly and I hate it.

**What you hope for...**

To experience greater peace with your body.

**What you say...**

Day by day I embrace the uniqueness of my body.

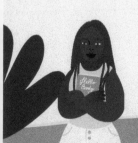

# Let's practice! Identify how you can practice bodacious body love by affirming your body.

### 1
What you see...

### 2
What you hope for...

### 3
What you say...

**1** What you see...

**2** What you hope for...

**3** What you say...

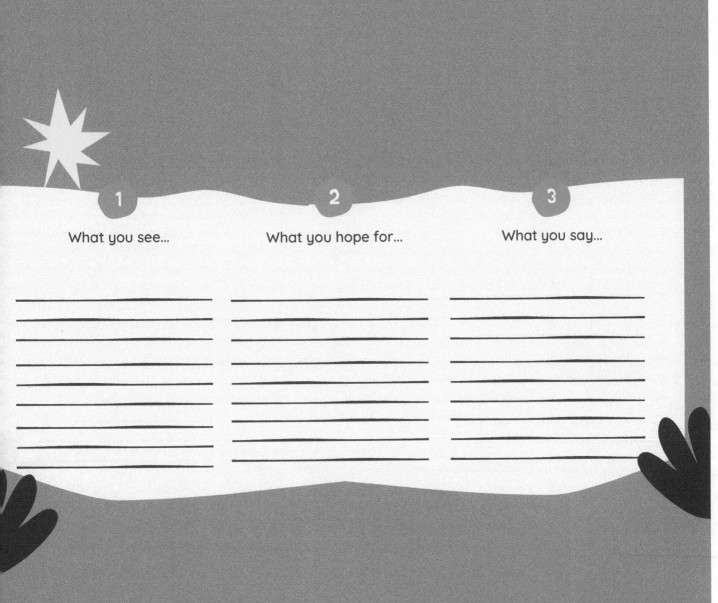

**1**

What you see...

_____
_____
_____
_____
_____
_____
_____
_____
_____

**2**

What you hope for...

_____
_____
_____
_____
_____
_____
_____
_____
_____

**3**

What you say...

_____
_____
_____
_____
_____
_____
_____
_____

**1** What you see...

_____
_____
_____
_____
_____
_____
_____
_____
_____

**2** What you hope for...

_____
_____
_____
_____
_____
_____
_____
_____
_____

**3** What you say...

_____
_____
_____
_____
_____
_____
_____
_____
_____

# Temperature Check

Rate how today's activity affected your mood.

If you are not where you'd like to be today, are there activities you may be able to engage in to assist you with improving your mood?

**HINT**:
Now would be a great time to add to your brag list.

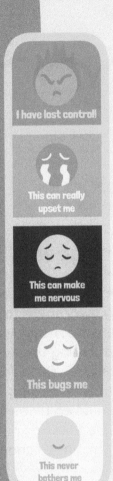

# Day Nineteen

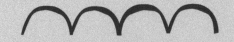

# Mirror Mirror

## You knew it was coming, here goes....

Set a timer for the amount of time you are able to safely tolerate. Stand in the mirror and look at yourself. Bring awareness to the thoughts that automatically creep into your consciouness. Write them down. Notice what feelings these thoughts bring up. Write them down. Be sure to breathe through this exercise. Consciously choose to practice self-compassion and grace by rewording the judgements you hold about yourself. Write them down below also. It may be helpful to complete this activity multiple times as needed and increase the amount of time as your mind begins to change about your body perception.

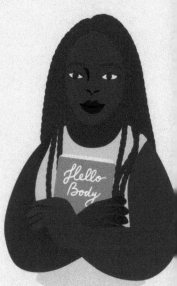

Notice your experience with today's activity.

Describe what went well and/or was challenging.

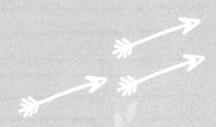

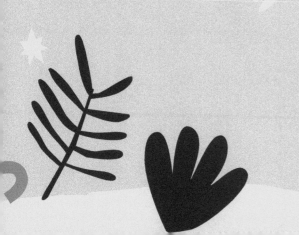

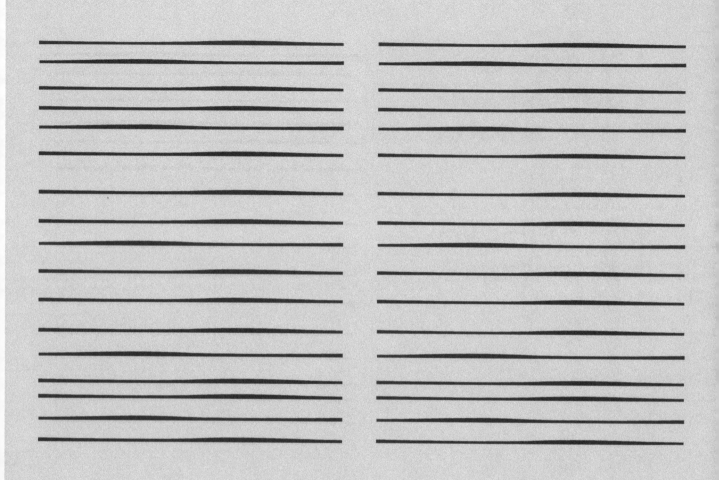

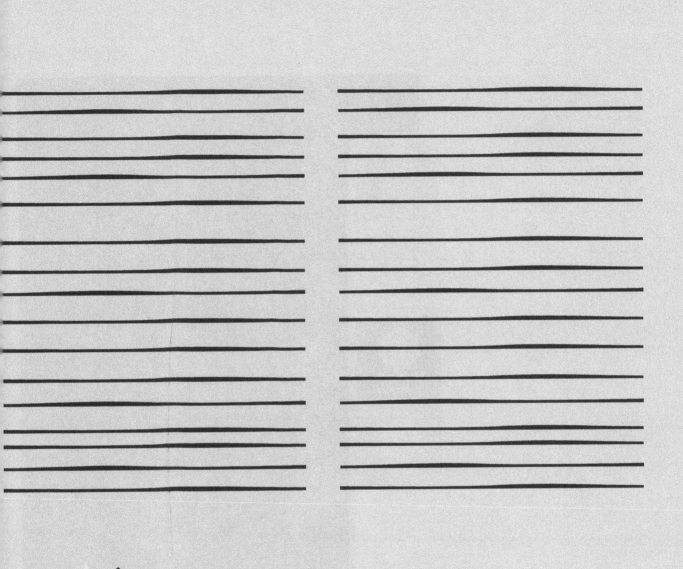
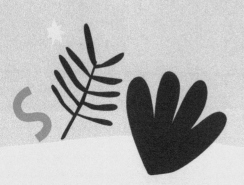

# Temperature Check

Rate how today's activity affected your mood.

If you are not where you'd like to be today, are there activities you may be able to engage in to assist you with improving your mood?

**HINT**:
Now would be a great time to add to your brag list.

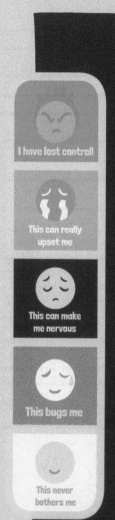

I have lost control!

This can really upset me

This can make me nervous

This bugs me

This never bothers me

# Day Twenty
## Fierce COdE:
## permission to be fierce

A code can be defined as words or phrases that communicate an attitude or meaning.  From this day forward I welcome you to the fierce girl club.  In this club we give ourselves permission to be exactly who and how we are...
without false humility,
with explanation,
without apology
and certainly without the need for external validation
We are the truest representative of the queen our Creator made us to be.

Allow your bodacious body love to be experienced by the world.  Purposely dress fierce...pull out that red lippie, that dress and those heels you spent wayyyy too much on...slip them on and flaunt your stuff, purposely.

Bonus if you take a selfie to clarify exactly who you are!!

Humor me a little!!
Free yourself to be fully who you are...all of you, in your own words!!

I, _____, give myself permission to BE:

_____

_____

In the fierce girl club we get to create our own body rules.

Describe your own fierce girl club rules.

How do you see yourself living your rules out?

# Temperature Check

Rate how today's activity affected your mood.

If you are not where you'd like to be today, are there activities you may be able to engage in to assist you with improving your mood?

**HINT**:
Now would be a great time to add to your brag list.

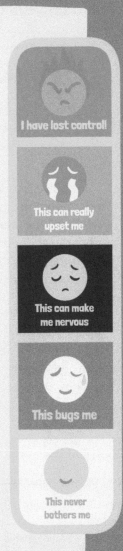

# Day Twenty-One

## You made it to bodacious body love!!!

You've journaled your way through gaining a greater understanding of your body image and the factors that play(ed) a role in how you see and speak to your body. You've learned how to shift your thinking to change how you interact with yourself. You've become requainted with your body and bodaciously chose to be your fierce self.

How will your life be different now? What supports can you set up for yourself to keep on track as you practice being mindful and intentional about your thought life and speaking the things your body needs to hear in your own voice rather than those of others or your inner critic?

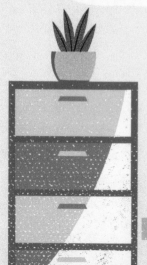

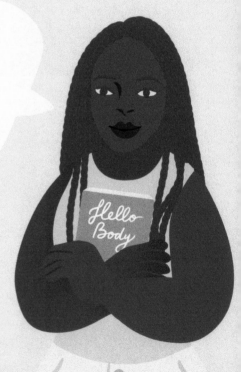

# Temperature Check

Rate how today's activity affected your mood.

If you are not where you'd like to be today, are there activities you may be able to engage in to assist you with improving your mood?

**HINT**:
Now would be a great time to add to your brag list.

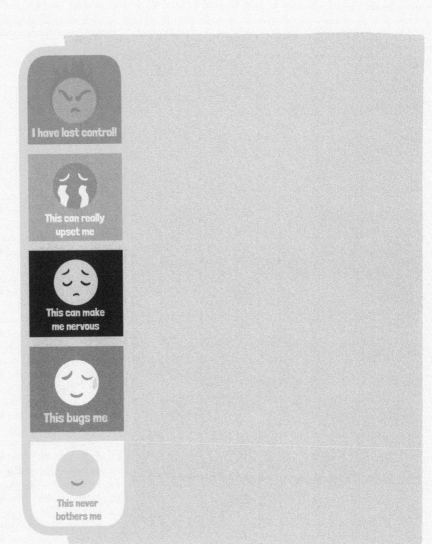

I have lost control!

This can really upset me

This can make me nervous

This bugs me

This never bothers me

This page
intentionally left
blank